MW01264645

Become

A

Physical

Therapist

Skip Hunter, PT, ATC
and
Lori Whitlow

SHE
Skip Hunter Enterprises, Inc.

Skip Hunter Enterprises, Inc.
PO Box 61
Clemson, SC 29633

Hunter, Skip
    How to become a physical therapist/Skip Hunter and Lori Whitlow
    — First Edition

ISBN 0-9649873-0-9

Library of Congress Catalog Number 95-95046

Page layout, typesetting, and cover design
by
Buster Kennedy

DEDICATION

This book is dedicated to all the "volunteer" students who have taken the time to spend their valuable hours observing in this labor of love we call Physical Therapy. All that we have done is show the love we feel toward a profession that has to be the greatest job in the world. Any experience shared with students is simply being passed on by the great teachers and therapists who shared this same experience with us. We hope that these volunteers will pass on the same enthusiasm when they become Physical Therapists. Although the road to school is long, stay the course. A wonderful occupation awaits you.

I dedicate this book to my dad, Stuart Hunter, Sr. His work ethics and approach to life have been my inspiration. From the first time he took me fishing, to his understanding of my escapades in high school and college, he has always been there for me. December 20, 1995 he told me, "Every day ends in darkness, but there is always light the next morning." Thanks for being there when I needed you, Dad.

Writing a book can be a great catharsis for life's problems. To my family, friends, and families of friends, I apologize for any burdens caused by my actions. You really can't get there from here–you have to go somewhere else to start.

"I'm not a very smart man." – Forest Gump, 1994

Skip Hunter, PT, ATC

This book is dedicated to my parents, Jim and Christine Whitlow, who have supported and encouraged me through the years. I love you Mom and Dad.

Lori Whitlow

ACKNOWLEDGEMENTS

Buster Kennedy, Ellen Bagwell, Jessica Milosch, Ed Raines, Lori Becker Jim Blanton, Jim Whitlow, Christine Whitlow, Alex Siffri, Lori Lanier, Lew G., Benette Barrus, Jennifer Coyne, Flora Riley, Jeb Hunter, Clay Hunter, Jane Hunter, Neil Richardson, and Ric Garcia.

The Average Physical Therapist

In a study by Pearl (1991) 416 Physical Therapist responded to a questionnaire about their career choice. Twenty-six percent were men and seventy four percent were women. Their average age was thirty-four. Sixty-six percent were married and forty-two percent had children. Eighty-one percent had a bachelors degree as their highest degree, sixteen percent had a masters, and three percent had Ph.D. The mean salary of this group was $34,790. Seventy-one percent of the average day was spent in patient care, while twenty-seven percent was spent in administrative duties.

Minorities in Physical Therapy

Although minorities currently make up twenty-four percent of the entire population, less than nine percent of the workers in the Physical Therapy profession belong to a minority. According to the Bureau of Labor Statistics, blacks account for eleven percent of the total work force, yet only three percent of Physical Therapist are black. Lack of information about Physical Therapy, low numbers of minorities in Physical Therapy education, and lack of financial assistance at the masters degree level are a few of the reasons given to account for this low percentage of minorities.

The Job Market

The physical therapy job market is hot! In a recent issue of the P.T. Bulletin there were 176 classified ads for Physical Therapist. These were located in nearly every section in the United States. The average salary for those jobs that listed a salary was $ 49,000 and many listed lucrative sign on bonuses between $1,000–$ 5,000.

Weekly and monthly Physical Therapy publications are filled with ads for Physical Therapists. The job market is so competitive that many job sites are now offering tuition reimbursement to Physical Therapy students who will sign on to work before they are enrolled in a Physical Therapy program. Others offer to pay back student loans or give lucrative sign on bonuses to attract therapists. Many of the large Physical Therapy companies offer to pay all or part of tuition costs if the potential student will agree to return and work for this company following graduation from a Physical Therapy program.

References

Conlan, B.J. Reconstruction Aides– Forerunners of modern PTOs. *Advance for Physical Therapist.* 5: pg. 8, 1994.

Currier, Dean. *Elements of Research in Physical Therapy.* Baltimore, Md. Williams and Wilkens, 1981, 3– 5.

Jones, Linda. PT– Related Associations Useful for Networking with Those Who Share. *Advance for Physical Therapy.* 28: 22– 23, 1994.

Murphy, J. Population of minority PTs must increase. *Advance for Physical Therapists.*25: 6, 1994.

Pearl, M.J. Factors Physical Therapist use to Make Career Decisions. *Journal of the American Physical Therapy Association.*70: 105– 107, 1990.

Sheestack, Robert. *Handbook of Physical Therapy.* 3rd Edition. Springer Publishing Company, New York, NY. 1977.

Tucker, James. Employment Ads. *PT Bulletin.* 10: 28– 70, 1995.

CHAPTER 2

Pre Physical Therapy

Pre Physical Therapy Preparation

The most important factors for acceptance into a Physical Therapy program is grades, grades, and grades. In a study by the faculty at the University of Miami, the major predictors of success in a Physical Therapy curriculum were undergraduate grade point average and prerequisite grade point average. Rheault and Shafernich-Coulson (1988) found a significant correlation between preprofessional grades and professional grades. This agrees with Balogun, Karacoloff and Farina (1986) who stated that preprofessional grade point average was the best predictor of academic performance in Physical Therapy school.

For those of you whose grade point average is not in the ozone, there are arguments which can be made if asked in an interview about your grades. Rheault and Shafernich–Coulson found that there was no significant correlation between preprofessional GPA and clinical performance. Clinical performance is what Physical Therapy is all about. A good point to make is "Shouldn't there be another way for admission committees to analyze a student's future clinical performance rather than solely using the preprofessional Grade Point Average?"

Most schools decide on which student to interview based on

grades and scholastic aptitude test or graduate record exam scores. These grades usually consist of the students overall grade point average and science grade point average. Someone with an overall grade point average of 3.0 and an average science grade point average of 3.4 may be attractive at one particular Physical Therapy program and not at another. It is important to find out from the school which grades interest them.

High School Preparation

The most important aspect of high school, as far as Physical Therapy is concerned, is a firm educational basis on which to build. Good grades are not a matter of luck as many would have you think, but hard work. The work ethic is important because it will carry over to your college career.

Learning how to use the library may be the most important lesson one learns in high school. Not only is the library a necessary place to find reference materials, it may be the only quiet place to study. Learn to dig for information. Many of the newer problem based learning programs look for students who have not been spoon fed in high school or college. These programs require students to find information on their own and apply it to problems or situations which they will encounter in the practice of the profession.

Many of the courses which are required in high school are the courses that will prepare you to excel in the same type of course in college. This means taking courses such as chemistry, physics, biology, and mathematics (calculus and algebra). If you are currently in high school, you should take time to look over the list of core courses required by many Physical Therapy schools. These will give you a good idea of the courses you should prepare to take as you enter college. You will find these listed later on in this chapter as prerequisites for Physical Therapy.

Take advanced level courses which challenge you. Be careful that should you take advanced placement for college credit, that you

A. Remember that the most important aspect of acceptance into Physical Therapy school is grades. It is better to take a course in high school and repeat it in college and make an A than take that same course in high school for college credit and make a B. Be sure if you exempt a course and qualify to start at a higher level that you are ready to make an A at that level. Often it is advisable to avoid skipping the lower level courses and make an A in these courses before advancing to higher level courses.

One of the hardest parts of being a graduating high school senior is deciding on a college major. If you are considering Physical Therapy as a career choice it is never too early to explore the profession. Take the time to visit a local Physical Therapy clinic and observe. Most clinics are very receptive to volunteers and will be glad to have you visit. While there have a list of career questions to ask the therapist. If your school has a career fair or career day, ask that a Physical Therapist be invited. Your school guidance counselor will be glad to assist you in any of these endeavors.

Early foundations are important in education. The basics which are taught in high school will eventually be used in Physical Therapy. Research your career ideas as thoroughly as possible to ease the transition into college.

Where to go to Undergraduate School to apply to PT school

The more prestigious the school the higher the chances of being accepted to PT school. This is of course if your grades are acceptable from wherever you go to school. If you go to a school as an undergraduate and there is a PT school located at this school, this may be an advantage. The obvious closeness of the PT school may allow you to make contact more often with the faculty and representatives who will eventually choose each new incoming class. The more recognizable your face and resume, often the more likely you are to be accepted.

Prerequisites for Physical Therapy Programs

There are no absolute requirements for all schools. Each school sets its own prerequisites. The following list is a compilation of the most commonly required courses by most schools. **You should write each school you are interested in to get a current list of requirements.**

Biology   8 semester hours

Chemistry   8–12 semester hours
    Often includes Organic Chemistry

Math (algebra or higher)   3 semester hours

Statistics   3 semester hours

Physics   8 semester hours

Anatomy/Physiology   8 semester hours
    May be taken as separate courses

Human Anatomy or Human Physiology
    Take this course late in college so that it is fresh in your
    memory during your first year of Physical Therapy school.

Psychology   9 semester hours
    Includes: Abnormal Psychology

Developmental Psychology

Sociology   3 semester hours

Speech   3 semester hours

English composition   6 semester hours

Computer Science   3 semester hours

Social Sciences   6–9 semester hours
    May include: political science
                     anthropology
                     other psychology
                     sociology

Humanities and Fine Arts   6–12 semester hours
    May include: foreign language
                     religion
                     history
                     art
                     music
                     literature
                     philosophy

Some schools require additional courses from a variety of disciplines. These courses can include:

Philosophy/Logic
Medical Ethics
Medical Terminology
Excercise Physiology
Microbiology
Exercise Physiology
Kinesiology
Technical Writing
Genetics
CPR
First Aide
Research Methods

References

Balogun, J., Karacoloff, L., Fabrina, N. Predictions of academic achievement in Physical Therapy. *Physical Therapy.* 66: 976-980, 1986.

Hayes, S.H., Block, A., Cade, W.T. and Skolsky, R. Examining Predictor Variables in the Physical Therapy Admissions Process-What Predicts Success in an Educational Program?: Poster Presentation. 1994 Joint Congress of Canada Physiotherapy Association and American Physical Therapy Association. *Physical Therapy.* 74: 510, 1994.

Rheault, W. and Shaferich-Coulson, E. Relationship between academic achievement and clinical performance in a Physical Therapy program. *Physical Therapy.* 68: 378-380, 1988.

CHAPTER 3

Applying to Physical Therapy School

Types of Physical Therapy Programs

There are PT programs that you can be accepted into straight out of high school. Upon acceptance you must maintain a certain grade point average your first two years of college to continue through the Physical Therapy program. Other programs require at least a bachelor's degree from a college for possible selection into PT school. This may be entry into either another bachelor's program or into a graduate level curriculum.

The first graduate level PT program was established at Case Western Reserve University in 1960. In 1979 the APTA House of Delegates voted to have all entry level PT programs to be postbaccalaureate by 1991. This has not happened although Physical Therapy education is moving toward a master's degree level curriculum as an entry level. Forty-eight percent of the entry level programs in 1993 were at the graduate level. This movement toward a postbaccalaureate degree is the obvious move of the future in Physical Therapy.

What difference does having an advanced degree such as a master's versus a bachelor's make? Research has shown that therapists with advanced degrees do not find jobs any easier or at any higher salary range. The advantage appears that therapists with advanced degrees rise to supervisory levels sooner and are more confident about taking on responsibility or leadership.

officers; they are in charge of scheduling interviews, they may indirectly influence acceptance or rejection just by their attitude. In other words they are extremely important individuals. Identify these gatekeepers early in the admission process and cater to them. A smile and a kind word may be worth a thousand letters of recommendation. This is particularly important when having phone conversations with these individuals.

The Application

The average application costs about $50–100 to file. This will obviously limit the number of applications you can send in. Send in only those that fit the following criteria:

- You have completed all the requirements for admission.

- You meet all the admissions standards.

- Location and finances fit both interview budget and the school budget. Keep in mind that the airfare to schools far away may be over $1000.

Once you have sent in your application, most schools advise strongly that you do not phone them to inquire as to your status. This obviously limits the large number of calls they would experience if this were allowed. Even if you do not call to inquire about your status, you should phone to make sure that your application is complete. This insures that the school does not disregard your application and blame it on some missing part of the paperwork. Be sure to get the name of the person you are speaking with if you are told that your application is complete.

Experience

Get a variety of experiences. Spend your summers keeping the hours a therapist keeps, working and or volunteering as a PT aide. Spend as much time as you can at these different sites. Don't be just another observer. Ask questions and get involved in the activities of the facility. The better you know the therapist, the more likely they will be willing to write a good recommendation letter for you in the future. If you are unable to volunteer in a Physical Therapy clinic, try to spend some time at a healthcare setting. Any healthcare life experience will be an asset on the application or in the interview.

Recommendation Letters

Know your references and make sure they are all of the same quality. A bad reference can bring questions to your abilities and greatly hurt your chances of getting an interview. Most schools will look favorably on letters from therapists. A letter from anyone connected with the school either as faculty or student will be of great value also.

Terminology

In interviews and essays, there is often asked a question based on the understanding of certain terms used in medicine and Physical Therapy. Following is a list of terms and definitions often used in Physical Therapy:

Range of Motion (ROM)   The amount of movement available in a joint.

Direct Access   Allowing a patient to enter into Physical Therapy treatment without referral from another practitioner.

Peer Review   Examination of clinical practice by someone of equal rank or status.

Functional Outcome Assessment   The ability of an individual to perform daily and real life activities after the conclusion of therapy.

ADA- Americans with Disabilities Act   A wide ranging piece of legislation which requires reasonable accommodation to an injured or handicapped worker by a place of employment. Established in 1991.

Managed Care   Payment systems that integrate the financing and delivery of health care to covered individuals with select providers.

Geriatrics   Sudy of all aspects of treatment of the aging/elderly.

Pediatrics   Study of all aspects of treatment on children.

Isokinetics   Exercise equipment which allows exercise to be performed at a constant velocity throughout the range of motion. Most of these machines are computer driven and are able to compare the strength of an injured limb against the strength of an uninjured limb.

PT Assistants   They work under the direct supervision of the PT. Responsible for assisting in treatment plans, conducting treatments and training patients.

Activity of Daily Living (ADL)   The self care, communication, and mobility required for independence in everyday living.

POPTS –Physician Owned PT Service   The APTA is opposed to situations in which physical therapists are employed or under agreement with referring practitioners in which the referring practitioner receives compensation either directly or indirectly for referring or prescribing Physical Therapy.

Manual Therapy   Therapy that is performed by mobilizing, massaging, or manipulating with the hands.

HMO- (Health Maintenance Organization)   Pay system in which the patient may be treated only by providers who belong to the organization.

PPO (Preferred Provider Organization)   Pay system in which the patient is given a fee reduction for having treatment by a member of the organization.

Workers Compensation   Insurance that provides pay and medical coverage should a worker be injured while performing their job.

Resources

The more you know about Physical Therapy, the easier the interview process will be. It will be to your advantage to read about Physical Therapy in several different publications.

The *Journal of the American Physical Therapy Association* is published monthly. Currently in its seventy third year, it is a scientific journal consisting of research pertinent to the field. Although most of the articles will be too in-depth for the average pre-Physical Therapy student, it is worthwhile to look over a copy to familiarize yourself with the leading journal of Physical Therapy.

Other publications which might be of value are The *PT Bulletin* which is a weekly publication by the APTA. This newspaper has feature stories on various aspects of Physical Therapy, seminar information, job openings, and interesting letters to the editor. The section on faculty openings in this bulletin is a good place to find programs which are just opening and are in the process of hiring new faculty. Applications to these schools often do not compete with as many other applications as older schools. Another section which is informative is the letters to the editor section. Often this section will have letters which contain many of the controversial subjects currently at the forefront of the physical therapy profession. This magazine may be subscribed to through the APTA.

Advance for Physical Therapist is another weekly Physical Therapy newsmagazine. It is published by Merion Publications, 650 Park West, King of Prussia, Pa. 19406–4025. It is similar in format to The *PT Bulletin* in that it contains articles, ads, and seminar information.

Most of the articles are more clinical in nature than those in The *PT Bulletin.*

Physical Therapy Forum is another publication of Merion Publications. This small booklet is published every two weeks and is mainly an employment opportunity magazine. It lists job openings and salaries by states. This is not a bad place to look to get some idea of just how hot the Physical Therapy market is.

Most of the sections of the APTA publish some type of magazine or newsletter. A good example of this is *The Journal of Orthopedic and Sports Physical Therapy* published by the Sports Medicine Section and the Orthopedic Sections of the APTA. This is an excellent clinical magazine with many good articles on the treatment of various sports and orthopedic problems.

You should familiarize yourself with these magazines and newsletters before your interview. Often the interviewer will ask some question which tests your knowledge of current Physical Therapy controversies and topics. Browsing through articles in these publications will help should you have to discuss any of these.

Tests

Many schools give some type of intelligence test on the day of the interview. Some examples of this are: word association or a personality test.

Many schools require that a standardized test be taken before applying to the school.

SAT – Scholastic Aptitude Test

The SAT test is taken by all high school students in the United States wishing to enter college. A majority of Physical Therapy freshman entry and bachelor's programs use the SAT as part of their ranking system. To be competitive for entry to Physical Therapy school, it is recommended that a minimum of 500 out of 800 be scored on each section. It is obvious that a high score on the SAT greatly improves your chances for admission to a good college. The SAT is a three hour examination given four times a year. It is made up of two sections:

Verbal – opposites, sentence completions, analogies and reading comprehension questions. This section measure your ability to read with comprehension and to deal with word and thought relationships.

Quantitative/Math – simple math, algebra, and geometry. This section measures your reasoning as well as your mathematical abilities.

To obtain a registration packet for the SAT write:

The College Board
2970 Clairmont Rd
Suite 250
Atlanta, GA   30329–1639
(404)–636–9465

ACT –American College Testing

The ACT is similar to the SAT and is taken by high school students. The ACT is a three hour test which examines ability in the fields of English, mathematics, social studies, and the natural sciences. The ACT test is a newer test which is used most often by smaller schools. These schools are located more often in the mid-west and South rather than the larger schools in the East which favor the SAT.

To obtain a registration packet for ACT contact:

American College Testing
2201 North Dodge Street
PO Box 168
Iowa City, IA   52243
(319)–337–1000

GRE–Graduate Record Exam

The GRE is considered by Physical Therapy programs as a way of evaluating likely success in graduate school. College students wishing to enter graduate school usually take the GRE between their junior and senior years. We feel that the sooner you take this standardized test after your basic math and English courses, the fresher this material will be to you.

It may be of benefit to take this test near the end of your sophomore year or at least near the start of the junior year. To be competitive for entry in to a Physical Therapy program, 500 out of 800 on each section is considered the minimum score by many schools. As with the SAT, the higher your score, the greater your chances for admission.

The GRE is a three hour exam given several times a year. It is divided into three sections:

Verbal   Analogies, antonyms, sentence completion, and reading comprehension

Quantitative   Arithmetic, algebra, geometry, data analysis, quantitative comparison, and problem solving

Analytical   Analytical reasoning, logical reasoning

The GRE is considered a vital part of many of the master's and Ph.D. Physical Therapy programs ranking system. The cost of the GRE is $56.00. To get a registration packet write:

Graduate Record Examinations
Educational Testing Service
PO Box 6004
Princeton, NJ 08541–6108
(609) –771–7670

You may also call:

609-921-9000
609-734-9362 Hearing Impaired
510-654-1200 Bay Area, CA
609-771-7670 Princeton, NJ

AHPAT – Allied Health Professions Admission Test

The AHPAT is a three and one-half hour test science and math test. This test is used as part of the admissions process by schools offering post-baccalaureate and baccalaureate degrees in allied health, i.e. Physical Therapy. The test is made up of five content areas:

Verbal Ability   Synonyms and antonyms; seventy-five questions

Quantitative Ability   Algebra, geometry, and basic trigonometry; fifty questions

Biology   Cell biology, heredity, human structure and function, bacteria and viruses, evolution and plants; fifty questions

Chemistry   Atoms and molecules, formulas, equations, bonding, element and periodic relationship, states of matter, acids, bases, electrochemistry, kinetics, and nuclear/organic chemistry; fifty questions

Reading Comprehension   Comprehension analysis, interpreting reading passages dealing with science-oriented topics; fifty questions

Cost of the AHPAT is $35.00. To get a registration packet write:

Allied Health Professions Admission Test
The Psychological Corporation
555 Academic Court
San Antonio, TX 78204-2498
or call: 512-921-8794

The Interview

Once the applications have gone in, many schools will take the top fifty to one hundred applicants to interview. Many times the interview can make or break an applicant. This can not be stated strongly enough. Often by the time the interviews are scheduled, grades are disregarded and the entire admission process hinges on the interview.

There is no doubt that practice enhances ones interviewing skills. We have listed several ideas and concepts based on the interviews of other previous applicants which may help you practice for this process.

What to Wear

Remember that the fifteen to forty-five minutes you spend with the interviewer may be the only look that the school gets of you. For men a coat and tie are mandatory. This does not necessarily mean a suit but a sport coat and tie at least. For women, a dress or suit of a conservative nature will be sufficient. It is important to be well groomed. This does not mean that you need a crew cut or excessive makeup, but that you should appear professional. Most PT schools when asked what they want in a PT applicant state that they are looking for someone who has professional potential.

What to Expect on the Day of the Interview

Most schools bring in some portion or all of the applicants to interview on one day or on several consecutive weekends. This allows the school to invite the interviewers as few times as possible. When you first get to the interview site, usually all the applicants to be interviewed will be gathered to detail what will happen the rest of the day. Afterwards, all applicants will be divided among interviewers, essay sites, and testing sites.

The Interviewers

The composition of the interview committee at different schools varies. Some schools use only faculty, while others will have students and outside therapists on the interview staff. If you are not told what the composition of the interviewing group is, then ask. It is important to know who you are talking to.

Some schools will have a single interviewer, while others may have as many as five individuals who interview a single applicant. Occasionally interviews are done as a group. Several people ask questions to a group of interviewees. Often in interviews where more than one person is interviewing, the interviewers will take on roles as friendly or adversary in order to see how you might handle stress. The interviewer whose job it is to stress you can throw out some intimidating questions to see how you react. Don't be afraid to admit that you are nervous. Its only human. Also don't be afraid to admit that you don't know the answer to a question or that you need a question clarified.

A new technique used by some schools is an interaction group, where a group of applicants is given a medical problem to problem solve openly in front of a panel of interviewers. This is particularly common in schools where independent learning is stressed. The major focus in this technique is to observe leadership and problem solving in a group situation.

An example of this is five students are brought in front of a panel of interviewers and told to discuss how to ration Physical Therapy services among a group of patients who have terminal illness, no insurance, no job versus a group of patients who have minor illness, good insurance, and good jobs.

Essay and Interview Questions

Since the essay may be the only look that an admissions committee may have of you, it is imperative that this writing present you in the best way possible. Something in your essay has to state that you are a unique individual e.g. you are different in a good way from those other 800 applicants! There are many books which may help you prepare for this task. A purchase of one of these how to books may be a wise investment. Once you have organized and prepared, it is advisable to write, rewrite, and rewrite until you are satisfied with the result. There are several things we feel that are important to keep in mind in writing your essay:

● Be positive. Do not use the essay format to explain why you did not do well on the SAT or GRE or chemistry.

● Get the readers attention early. Dare to be different by starting the essay differently or stating a fact about yourself that will leave the reader wanting to read more. Remember the interview committee will read hundreds of these essays.

● If your essay is on a subject other than yourself, make sure to research the topic thoroughly.

● Develop a line of thought and follow through with it in the essay. Your last paragraph should package up the entire thought.

● Keep it short and simple.

● Be yourself and communicate confidence.

● Find someone with literary knowledge to look at what you have written and give you an honest opinion about it.

We have found that the easiest way to prepare for either interview or essay questions is to practice by writing down the answers to questions which might be asked. Even if the questions are not exactly the same, the answers to some of the following questions might be useful in your interview or essay.

Following is a list of possible interview and essay questions which have been popular in the past. Look over these and write down what your answer would be.

- Most embarrassing moment.

- What was your proudest moment?

- Do you have an area you would like to specialize in?

- Tell me about yourself.

- What is the most important social issue of our times?

- Why do you think we should let you in instead of the other candidates?

- Why did you make a C in chemistry?

- Who do you admire most?

- What has been the hardest moment in your life.?

- What are your weak points / strong points?

- What color best describes you?

- If you were a car what kind would you be?

- What will you be doing five years from now. In ten years?

- Worst semester you had and why?

- What do you know about the APTA?

- Have you done any research?

(interview and essay questions continued)

- Why did you choose PT over your current profession?

- Main reason PT uses patient goals.

- Best place you observed and why?

- Worst place you observed.

- Other than direct patient contact what roles/responsibilities do PTs take on?

- How do you feel your undergraduate degree will help you in PT?

- Important issues facing PT.

- What do you think of PTAs roles?

- What are your hobbies?

- What do you do in your free time?

- Biggest failure and how you handled it.

- Why do you want to become a PT?

- Why do you think you will make a good PT?

- What will you do if you don't get in?

- What do you think of HMOs and managed care?

- What do you hate?

- Is there an advantage to being a DPT or MPT over a bachelor's?

- Do you think direct access is good or bad?

- What do you least like about PT?

- How do you learn best?

- How do you relieve stress?

- What do you consider a stressful situation?

- Why did you choose our school?

- How will you balance being a PT with your social / family life?

- What do you think of the Health Care plans which are being discussed?

- If you could be anyone who would it be?

- How do you handle criticism?

- Tell us about your leadership qualities.

- If you had all the money in the world what would you do?

References

AHPAT, The American Psychological Corporation, Harcourt Brace Jovanovich, Inc. 1992: 26–27.

Barr, J., A problem solving curriculum design in Physical Therapy. Doctoral Dissertation. Chapel Hill, NC University of North Carolina, 1975.

Barr, Jean S., *Planning Curricula in Physical Therapy*, Section for Education, APTA, Feb. 3,4,5, 1976: 54–55.

Burnett, C., Mahoney, P., Chidley, M. and Pierson, F. Problem Solving Approach to Clinical Education. *Physical Therapy.* 66: 1730–1733, 1986.

General Test Descriptive Booklet 1994–1995, Educational Testing Service, 1994: pg. 3.

Reichley, M.L. MPT degree creep. *Advance for Physical Therapist.* 21: 21, 1995.

Warren, S.C. and Pierson, F.M. Comparison of characteristics and attitudes of entry-level bachelor's and master's degree students in Physical Therapy. *Journal of the American Physical Therapy Association.* 74: 333–348, 1994.

CHAPTER 4

The Average
Applicant

The 1994 Applicant Report

In 1991 The American Physical Therapy Association began to collect
data on applicants to Physical Therapy schools in an effort to find out
more about who was applying to the profession. Schools were asked
to send a questionnaire to it's pool of applicants. Schools were
allowed to identify applicants. Some schools considered an applicant
to be anyone who asked for an admission application, while other
schools only questioned those students who filled out and completed
an application. Although all of the accredited programs in the United
States were asked to participate, not all programs agreed to do so. In
1992–93 eighty-five programs participated, while in 1994–95 eighty-six
participated. This represented 5,133 applicants who returned the form.
The rest of this chapter are statistics taken directly from the 1994
Applicant Report.

The Competition

Age   The largest percentage of applicants (57.9%) were between the
ages of 21–25. The next largest group according to age was between
the ages of 26–29 (22.3%). The remainder of the ages were younger
than 20 (5.6%), 30–39 (11.9%), and over 40 (2.6%). The mean age of
applicants in 1994 was 24.8 years.

Gender, Marital Status, and Ethnic Background   Females accounted for 69.3% of the applicants. 84.1% of the applicants were single. 11.2% of the those applicants applying to professional school belonged to a minority racial or ethnic group.

Residence   The largest percentage of applicants came from California (8.8%), New York (7.5%), Texas (6.5%), Pennsylvania (6.2%) and Illinois (5.4%).

Educational Background of Parents   26.0% of the fathers and 23.8% of the mothers of applicants had bachelor's degrees. 14.6% of the fathers and 11.3% of the mothers of applicants had master's degrees. 18.9% of the fathers and 26.0% of the mothers of applicants had high school diplomas. Only 4.6% of the fathers and 3.2% of the mothers did not finish high school.

Educational Backgrounds of Applicants   Only 1.4% of the applicants were Physical Therapy Assistants. Most of the applicants were in their senior year of college (58.7%). A large portion (23.2%) of the applicants were students who were pursuing prerequisite courses at the time of application. 24.4% of the applicants were majoring in some type of natural science, 16.3% were in pre-physical therapy, and 10.5% were in exercise/physical education in their undergraduate studies.

Grades   49.0% of the applicants had a GPA between 3.0–3.49. 36.5% had over a 3.5 Grade Point. Only 14.6% of the applicants had a cumulative GPA under a 3.0.

Standardized Test Scores   The SAT mean score was 489 verbal and 564 quantitative. 21% of the applicants made higher than 550 on the verbal and 55.6% made higher than 550 on the quantitative portion. Students who took the ACT test averaged 24.3 in 1994. GRE scores were 583 mean in quantitative, 489 in verbal, and 590 in analytical ability. 65.5% of the applicants who took the analytical part of the GRE scored higher than 550, 63.4% higher than 550 in quantitative, and 20.5% higher than 550 on verbal. Some schools require the Allied Health Professions Aptitude Test. The test is scored from 1 to 99 on verbal, biology, chemistry, quantitative, and reading. The means of scores reported were as follows: quantitative,71; verbal, 61.1; biology, 68.7; chemistry, 70.1; and reading, 64.3. The Miller Analogies test is a logic test which some schools give to perspective applicants. The average score on this test among applicants was 53.3.

Reapplying Students   28.9% of the applicants had previously applied for admission to a Physical Therapy program. This number is surprisingly high and indicates that many of the applicants who do not get in one year will reapply the following year.

Reasons applying to Physical Therapy school   66.5% of the respondents stated that the major reason for applying to Physical Therapy school was to help others. 57.% liked the variety that the Physical Therapy profession offers. 28.4% liked the physically active part of Physical Therapy. Keep these reasons in mind if you are asked to write about your choice of Physical Therapy as a career. Most individuals reading an essay on your career choice like to read a unique perspective.

How many programs did each respondent apply to   26.3% applied to 6–10 programs; 20.5% to 2–3; 20.0% to 4–5; 15.5% applied to only one.

References

Applicant Report-1994. The American Physical Therapy Association-Division of Research, Analysis, and Development. June 1995.

CHAPTER **5**

Conversations
With
Admissions Officers

Questions

In an effort to present the best possible view of exactly what most
Physical Therapy schools are looking for in a prospective student, we
contacted several of the individuals on admissions committees using a
cross section of large, small, private and public institutions. These
schools were representative of all parts of the United States. Each
person was asked the following questions:

1. Can we use your name and school name?

2. What are you looking for in a prospective student?

3. What red flags do you look for in the student who will not do
   well at your school?

4. What qualities enhance the chance of acceptance?

5. How much of the admissions process is grades vs. interview?

6. What are the components of your point system?

7. Do you have minimum GRE scores and GPAs that are acceptable?

Each of these individuals was asked to expand on any of the answers which needed further explanation. Interestingly there were several schools which would not answer these questions during a phone interview. The explanations for these refusals ranged from "I do not have the authority to release such information" to " our program is strictly an objective admissions. We take the scores, crunch the numbers, and admit the top twenty-four out of this process." Fortunately there were schools which gladly answered the questions and more.

Admissions Officer #1

Mike Gross, Ph.D., P.T.
Associate Professor
Chairman, Admissions Committee
University of North Carolina Chapel Hill
Chapel Hill, NC

What are you looking for in a Physical Therapy student? We are seeking a student who is academically capable; someone who has done their homework on the profession. We do not advise that a student spend a lot of time on one single environment within Physical Therapy as a volunteer, but to spend time in different areas. It should take a student no more than two days to figure out what goes on in a certain clinic or area of Physical Therapy. We advise that the student spend some quality time with a therapist to discuss issues facing the profession and to discuss the therapists work. We like students to experience the breadth of the profession.

What red flags do you look for in the student who will not do well in your program? The students who will not fare well in our program are not academically capable; they can not communicate in written form. We require several written essays. In these we look for insight into the profession, their strengths and weaknesses, and how these will help or hinder them.

What qualities enhance getting in? Academically capable; good written and oral communication skills. Knowledgeable regarding the profession, themselves, and how they fit with the profession; responsible,aware of the world around them.

How much of the admissions process is grades vs. interview? 48% of the admissions process is based on grades. The breakdown for this is:

1. Prerequisite GPA–This is the most important aspect of grades and is weighted twice the importance of the other grades.
2. GPA for the last two years of the baccalaureate degree.
3. GRE score is weighted the least of the academic criteria.

Fifty-two percent of the admissions process is based on the subjective rating of the applicant's written application and the interview.

Components of your point system. Given above

Do you have a minimum GRE or GPA? Yes. The graduate school has a minimum score on the GRE based on the cumulative scores of all three parts. The minimum GPA for the graduate school is a 3.0.

Admissions Officer # 2

Ellen Spake, M.S., P.T.
Director
Physical Therapy Program
Rockhurst College
1100 Rockhurst Road
Kansas City, Mo.   64110

What are you looking for in a Physical Therapy student? We are clearly looking for someone who is bright enough to be successful in a rigorous academic program but equally 1) knows enough about

Physical Therapy to make an informed decision and to be able to articulate why they are a good match for the profession. 2) has the communication skills to function well in the profession.

What red flags do you look for in a student who will not do well at your school? Anyone who does not have strong academics. A person who has not thoroughly investigated Physical Therapy as a profession. Someone who can't articulate why they are a good match for Physical Therapy in writing or orally. A person who does not exhibit good communication skills both verbal and non verbal.

Qualities which enhance chances of getting in. Excellent communication skills. We do not require an essay but do ask for a personal statement. Misspelled words and poor grammar are bad signs. Strong academics.

How much of the admissions process is grades vs. interview? 50% grades and 50% recommendation and interview.

Components of your point system. Cumulative GPA 15%, Science GPA 35%, Recommendation 30%, Interview 20% (subject to change)

Do you have a minimum GPA or GRE? The GRE is not required. The minimum GPA is listed as a 2.85 to apply. However meeting the minimum GPA may not qualify a student for an interview.

Admissions Officer #3

Robert Laird, Ph.D., PT
Graduate Program in Physical Therapy
North Georgia College
Barnes Hall, Room A-6
Dahlonega, GA   30597

What are you looking for in a Physical Therapy student? First, we need proof of academic ability. At North Georgia College there are two steps:

1. The student must be accepted into the Graduate school.
2. The student must be accepted into the Physical Therapy program.

What red flags do you look for in the student who will not do well at your school? The individual that does not finish. They may have many withdrawals on their transcript. They may have a history of switching around a lot. We look for individuals who can carry through; someone with consistency. Letters of recommendation and narrative responses may give insight to this.

What qualities enhance the chances of getting in? This is a complex answer. The individual must have the proper credentials on paper as well as the proper personal attributes.

How much of the admissions process is grades vs. interview? Grades are secondary once academic ability is proved. Grades and interview are not the only two things looked at; recommendation letters, essays, etc. are also looked at.

What are the components of your point system? We use a score sheet to tally before the interview. An individual gets points for overall GPA, Science GPA, GRE scores, evidence of leadership and recommendation letters. Grades and GRE are the largest share with leadership scored just below these. Points are tallied and the top 85 individuals are usually interviewed. The interview is scored and the two scores are added. Interviews are weighted more than the paper scores.

Do you have minimum GRE scores and GPAs that are acceptable? These are determined by the state of Georgia. They require a minimum of 400 on each section of the GRE and a minimum GPA of 2.7.

Admissions Officer # 4

Mr. Jim Youdas, M.S., P.T.
Chairman, Admissions Committee
Physical Therapy Program
Mayo School of Health Related Sciences
1105 Siebens Building
Rochester, Minnesota   55905

What are you looking for in a Physical Therapy student? The ideal
individual would have a 3.3 GPA or above, both science and overall.
The combined GRE scores would be at least 1500 or above. Observation
in Physical Therapy would be at least 100 hours, preferably not in one
area such as Sports Medicine.

*What red flags do you look for in the student who will not do well at
your school?* GPA below a 3.0. References which are bland or
critical. Individuals that have changed careers or been on a rocky
educational road and need to raise their GPA after graduation so they
go at night or take one science course per quarter to obtain a high
grade. This environment is not as intense as regular school and may
not be indicative of future performance.

Qualities which enhance chances of getting in. Four performance
skills are evaluated: verbal expression, problem solving, goal setting,
and interaction with people. Each individual is asked to retrieve
experiences from their own lives to show that they have these skills.

How much of the admissions process is grades vs. interview. 50%
grades and 50% interview. During the last application period 580
individuals applied, 150 were interviewed, and 36 were accepted. The
interviews are structured so that each person is interviewed by only
one team of two interviewers.

Components of your system. Grades, references, work experience or volunteer time accounts for a possible 20 points on our system. The interview accounts for a possible 16 points.

CHAPTER 6

What to Do
If You Are Accepted

Physical Therapy Curriculum

Although there are no absolute standards for Physical Therapy curriculums, there are traditional courses which are taught in most Physical Therapy programs whether the program is a masters level program or an undergraduate program. These courses may be assigned different credit hours by different schools according to the school's educational purpose. The first year of the educational program is usually spent in teaching the basic science and patient care courses to prepare the student for their residency or affiliation year(s) to follow. This affiliation time is spent in various settings of Physical Therapy to allow the student to practice the skills and techniques learned in the classroom setting. Most schools require a variety of settings for the affiliations to make sure the student receives a broad look and experience in the many facets of Physical Therapy.

First Year Courses

Basic Science

Gross Human Anatomy   This is usually the largest single credit hour course taken in the basic science curriculum. Body systems and regions are studied using dissection of human cadavers, prosected specimens, and skeletons. Classroom and laboratory sessions are used in teaching this course.

Histology   The study of microscopic tissue structure in the human body. Often this is studied at the cell level.

Medical Physiology   A study of body systems and how they interrelate. Often this study of physiological systems and principles is studied in relation to exercise and the effects of exercise on these systems.

Neuroanatomy   A detailed study of the structure and function of the central nervous system. Brain dissection and case studies are used to present this course.

Pathology   The study of disease and disease processes as related to different body systems.

Kinesiology   The application of biomechanical principles to movement of the body.

Functional Anatomy   Principles of biomechanics, physiology, and joint structure as applied to movement and function.

Patient Care Courses

Medical Communication (Medical Terminology)   The study of terms often used in Medicine as related to Physical Therapy. Also included in this course is instruction in writing and dictating medical notes for patients charts. Like many of the other medical fields, the amount of paperwork required to document patient care and treatments has become an increasing time constraint in Physical Therapy. Medical communication has become a very critical part of Physical

Therapy education due to both government regulations and insurance reimbursement.

Clinical Skills   This course may be subdivided into many different courses according to the school. However it is structured, it includes a study of all the various aspects of patient care needed by a therapist. This includes physical agents such as ice, heat, water, and modalities (electricity, ultrasound, massage, etc.). The use of exercise in the treatment of various disorders is also a major portion of this course. These types of courses are often the most enjoyable in the Physical Therapy curriculum since often the students only practice on each other before they actually perform the treatment on a patient.

Affiliations   Most schools require time spent in several different settings such as orthopedics, rehabilitation, neurology, pediatrics, burns, and geriatrics. These rotations or affiliations may last any length of time including days, weeks or even months.

Special Courses Offered in Master's Programs

Directed Research or Thesis Preparation   This course is the actual preparation of an independent project or significant research study presented in a thesis format . This requires vigorous scientific inquiry followed by utilization of writing skills.

Professional Issues   Many masters level programs and undergraduate programs offer a course dealing with ethics, health values, current controversies in Physical Therapy and healthcare in general. Professional organizations and relationships with other healthcare groups is also covered.

Finances

The money required to attend some Physical Therapy schools is staggering. Besides tuition, concern should be given toward books, housing, food, insurance, possible uniforms (lab jackets), immunizations, malpractice insurance, travel expenses to and from clinicals, housing at clinicals, and health insurance. The following list is the cost of certain schools from recent catalogs. If you are interested in any of these schools, contact the school financial office to request the most recent tuition and expense information.

University of Central Florida	$55.39 / credit hr. $218.80 / credit hr. $275 / semester	in-state out-of-state books
Chapman University	$385 / credit hr.	
Medical College of Georgia	$654 / quarter $1148 / quarter	in-state out-of-state
Midwestern University	$13,750 / year $15,750 / year	in-state out-of-state
Shenandoah	$13,000 / year	
North Georgia College	$6,320 $ 2,340	total books
Boston College	$18,420 / 9 months $770	books
Rockhurst College	$4,745/ semester $200–400	books
Slippery Rock	$8,000 / yearly $9,500 / yearly $550 / semester	in-state out-of-state books
Widener	$13,700 / yearly	

University of Evansville	$5900 / semester	
Temple University	$247 / credit hr.	in-state
	$333 / credit hr.	out-of-state
Philadelphia College of Pharmacy	$10,600 / yearly	tuition

Financial Aid

As one can see from the financial information given in the previous section, Physical Therapy school can be a costly adventure. Once costs of living: housing, utilities, food, insurance, are calculated into school costs such as tuition, books, and incidental expenses, a Physical Therapy education can amount to $50–60,000.

There are several ways to finance your education through the Federal Government loan program. The schools currently participating in the Federal Direct Loan Program number 1500. There are four different direct loans offered by the government:

1. **Federal Direct Stafford Loan** These loans are given according to financial need. The government pays all interest while the student is in school. The interest rate on this loan is variable and is adjusted each July. The maximum rate of interest will never be over 8.25 percent.

2. **Federal Direct Unsubsidized Stafford/Ford Loan** The government does not pay the interest while the student is in school. No financial need is required for this loan. The interest rate on this loan is also under 8.25 percent.

3. **Federal Direct PLUS Loans** These loans are given to parents with good credit who want to pay for their dependent students. The parents pay the interest for the student. The interest rate on this loan is also variable and will never exceed 9 percent.

4. Federal Direct Consolidation Loan This loan combines one or more federal loans into one new direct loan. Only one monthly payment is made.

How much you can borrow depends on your year in school, how long you will be in school, your school costs, how much your family will pay, and whether you classify as a independent or dependent student.

The total limits on subsidized loans is $23,000 for undergraduate and $65,500 for graduate study. The total limit on both subsidized and unsubsidized loans is $23,000 for undergraduate, $46,000 for an independent undergraduate student, and $138,500 for a graduate or professional student including loans for undergraduate study.

To apply for a Direct subsidized or unsubsidized loan, you must fill out a free application for Federal Student Aid. After this is given to your school, the school will determine the amount of your award and the type of loan best suited for you. You will then be required to sign a note stating that you will repay the loan. The school will either credit your account at the school with the amount of the loan or will pay you the amount by check. While you are enrolled in school at least half time you will not have to make payments on the loan. Six months after exiting school or dropping below half time enrollment you will need to start repayment of the loan. There are several options for repayment:

• A fixed payment over a fixed period of time of up to ten years.

• An extended repayment period of up to thirty years (requires more interest to be paid).

• A payment plan in which the payments gradually increase over time (especially useful for those whose income will increase as they work longer).

• A plan in which the payments are adjusted according to income. Your required monthly payment will not exceed twenty percent of your discretionary income.

Another method of federal assistance is the Pell Grant. Eligibility for this grant depends on the calculated family contribution, the cost of school, and status of the student. Funding of the program determines the amount of award. The maximum amount awarded in 1994 was $2,300. The federal Perkins loan is a low interest loan for students in great need of financial aid. In this case the college is the lender of the amount of the award. Students may borrow $3,000 a year and the repayment is over a ten year period. Under certain work conditions (teaching low income students, peace corps, etc.) the loan repayment may actually be canceled.

States also have financial aid programs for qualified students. Each state has its own set of regulations concerning loans. To find out if you qualify for a state loan in a certain state you should write the Student Loan Program of that particular state.

Private foundations and organizations offer financial aid to qualifying students. Often these funds are available according to your parents occupation, your interest, your religion, or other factors in your life.

If you have questions about financing your education, contact the financial aid office at your school. All the information needed to decide on a loan will be available at this location.

There are other ways to obtain money for Physical Therapy school. Often corporations or hospitals will offer education monies to students who are accepted into school provided the student will sign a contract agreeing to work for the loaning institution for a certain period of time. Some will even agree to pay the entire tuition in return for a certain period of employment by the prospective student. An example of this might be: Student A is accepted into Physical Therapy school. Corporation B needs Physical Therapists, therefore it offers Student A $5,000 per year for school in return for a guarantee that Student A will work for the corporation for two years following graduation after passing the Physical Therapy licensure exam.

References

All About Direct Loans. William D. Ford Federal Loan Program brochure.

Paying Less For College. Princeton, N.J. Petersons 12th edition, 1994.

CHAPTER 7

What to Do
If You Are
Not Accepted

Never, Never, Never Give Up
Winston Churchill, 1941

The first thing to do if you are not accepted to any of the schools you have applied to is do not take it personally. Remember that no matter where you applied, many individuals were competing for that same slot you were after. Have realistic expectations on your chances of admission. This will ease the pain if you are not accepted.

Once the initial shock of rejection is over, get down to business of ascertaining why you did not get in. Most schools will give you a reason why your application was not accepted. Phone the school and ask for the Director or the Admissions officer. Be nice, but firm on finding the answer to your question. Remember you may apply to the program again next year and this phone call may be start of that process.

Ways to Improve Your Chances

If you find that your application was weak in certain areas, there are ways to strengthen the weak area. The following ideas may be used to increase your chances if one particular area is weak:

GRE/SAT Scores   Scores on the SAT, GRE, ACT, and AHPAT cannot be overemphasized. Often these scores are counted just as much as your grade point.

There are courses which are given to help you prepare for these standardized tests. These review courses are designed to give you practice on questions which are similar to the ones given in the actual test. It is not uncommon for these courses to raise your score significantly if approached with diligence. There are also many books on the market which review the most commonly asked questions.

Both of these approaches will help only if you put the proper amount of work into them. There is no magical solution. Hard work and careful study will be the two methods which will eventually raise your test scores.

Grades   If your grade point average is too low, then you must take additional courses to raise it. It is important to find out from each school if the deficiency in GPA was in your overall or prerequisite GPA. Depending on the answer to this question, you should take either upper level prerequisite courses or just take additional courses which might raise your GPA. Find out from the schools you applied to if they will let you retake courses which you did not perform well in and count your new grade instead of the old grade. Often it is possible to take these courses at night and maintain a job during the day. Taking a course which is not required but is known as a particularly hard subject will sometimes impress an admissions committee. Organic chemistry, biochemistry, or an upper level biology course, such as genetics, may be viewed favorably if you score highly.

The important part of this formula is that you make good grades. Whatever you decide to take, it should result in an A. Remember that if you have all the required prerequisites, often the admissions committee looks only at your composite grade point, and not what courses you made those grades in.

Volunteer Experience   If the schools are not pleased with the amount of volunteer work performed then you may need to volunteer more hours or in different settings. Remember to vary your settings.

Some schools will favor individuals who have been exposed to a wide variety of Physical Therapy settings. This was mentioned in almost every interview with admissions officers.

In-state Residency Requirements   Some schools give a preference to instate residents. State supported schools will often only accept five to ten percent of each class as out of state residents. If you live in a state that has only one school while other states have several, you may think about moving and establishing residence in that state. It is important that you research this idea thoroughly since each state has its own residency requirements.

Letters of Recommendation   Unless you were able to read the recommendation given by an individual and it was outstanding, you should consider asking another person to write for you the next year. Physical Therapy schools will not inform you if your letters of recommendation were the cause of your non acceptance. Consider that the person you thought wrote you a good letter did not if there is no other good explanation why you were not accepted. Letters of recommendation should be enthusiastic, of moderate length, and well worded.

There is good news behind the let down of rejection. Most schools look favorably on individuals who are reapplying. This perseverance means something to those who judge which applicant should get in and which should not. Many schools will add points onto the rating scale of an individual who is reapplying for a second or third time. Be sure to emphasize that you are reapplying if you are. This may impress the admissions committee enough to strengthen your application.

   If Physical Therapy is what you want to do with your life, do not let rejections stand in your way but rededicate yourself to making your application stronger next time. Use this rejection to drive yourself even harder toward reaching your goal. Never, never, never give up!

CHAPTER 8

Physical Therapy Assistants

Defining the Role of
Physical Therapy Assistants

The Physical Therapy Assistant is a technical health care provider who works under the supervision of a licensed Physical Therapist. The responsibilities of the Physical Therapist Assistant (PTA) are to implement the plan of treatment as specified by the Physical Therapist. This includes exercises, modalities, recordkeeping and direct patient contact.

History of Physical Therapy Assistants

Physical Therapy Assistants (PTA) originated in the late 1940's because of the great shortage of therapists during the war and polio epidemic. In 1949 the APTA House of Delegates voted to acknowledge the need for therapy assistants. Until 1964 these assistants had little training other than on the job training. Catherine Worthington, Ph.D., PT, addressed the issue of training these assistants at the annual conference. The Board of Directors voted to form a committee to study the need for training of these non-professionals. As a result the APTA adopted the definition and policy currently used today for

PTA's. In 1970 the APTA extended affiliate membership to Physical Therapy Assistants.

The first two PT Assistant education programs began in 1967 at Miami Dade Community College in Florida and The College of St. Catherines in Minnesota. Currently there are over 130 Physical Therapy Assistants programs in the U.S. Most of these are located in the community or technical college system.

The need for Physical Therapy Assistants continues to grow just as the need for Physical Therapists continues to grow. There are currently 20,000 Physical Therapy Assistants in the United States. The Department of Labor and Statistics predicts that there will be a need for approximately 65,000 by the year 2000.

The competition to be accepted into Physical Therapy school is so great that many individuals who are turned down for Physical Therapy school will apply to Physical Therapy Assistants school. Other reasons may be financial, time constraints, and uncertainty about the career choice. There has been a recent trend toward Physical Therapy Assistants going on to Physical Therapy school after practicing as an assistant for a period of time. Barry University in Miami is one of several universities which have a weekend master's program in Physical Therapy for Physical Therapy Assistants.

Academic Requirements

Many of the Physical Therapy Assistant programs have admissions guidelines which are similar to those of Physical Therapy except on a lesser scale. Since the requirements for admission vary greatly from school to school, it is important to ask the schools you are interested in to send you a list of their requirements for admission. Most Physical Therapy Assistant schools have at least some of the following requirements:

• SAT or ACT scores which meet requirements. This is usually about 400 on each section of the SAT or 20 on each section of the ACT.

- Completion of certain developmental courses such as human anatomy and physiology, psychology, medical terminology, chemistry, and biology.

- Transcripts from all high school and colleges attended.

- Many schools require volunteer hours in a Physical Therapy setting.

- Some schools will interview prospective students.

Physical Therapy Assistant Curriculum

There are several different degree options for Physical Therapy Assistants. The school lasts two years and usually incorporates many of the basic collegiate math, English and elective courses normally taken as a freshman in college. The final year of Physical Therapy Assistants School teaches basic science and physical therapy courses along with clinical rotations to practice what has been taught. Listed below is a sample curriculum from Gwinnett Tech in Lawrenceville, Georgia for the class entering in the fall of 1994.

First Quarter
Human Anatomy and Physiology
General Psychology
Medical Terminology
CPR

Second Quarter
Human Anatomy and Physiology II
English Comp I
Humanities

Third Quarter
English Comp II
College Algebra
Oral Communication

Fourth Quarter
    Kinesiology
    Pathology
    Introduction to Patient Care Skills

Fifth Quarter
    Kinesiology II
    Pathology II
    Patient Care Skills II

Sixth Quarter
    Clinical Education I
    Patient Care Skills III
    Physical Therapy Seminar

Seventh Quarter
    Psychology of Adjustment
    Community Health and Welfare
    Patient Care Skills IV

Eighth Quarter
    Clinical Education II
    Clinical Education III
    (Gwinnett Technical Manual, 1994)

References

Adams, R.C. Physical Therapists Assistants change with the times. *Advance for Physical Therapists.* 4: 5–6, 1993.

Gwinett Technical Manual. The Physical Therapy Assistant. 1–24, 1994.

Murphy, J. PTAs brave bias to become PTs. *Advance for Physical Therapists.* 13: 4–5, 1995.

CHAPTER 9

Alphabetical Listing of Physical Therapy Schools in the US

Following is a list of the Physical Therapy schools in the United States as of 1994. Some of these programs may have been discontinued due to accreditation problems and others may have been added as a result of accreditation. The director of the schools program is listed after the name of the school. If you are interested in one of these schools check to be sure that the school is currently accredited, that the address is current, and that the head of the program has not changed since publication of this book.

Alabama

University of Alabama Birmingham
Marilyn Grossman, Ph.D., PT
Professor and Division Director
Division of PT
School of Allied Health Professions
UAB
SHRP Building, RM 116
Birmingham, AL   35294–1270
205–934–3566
Public university

University of South Alabama
Giovanni De Domenico, Ph.D., PT, Chair
Dept. of PT
University of South Alabama–Spring Hill Campus
1504 Spring Hill Avenue
Mobile, AL   36604
334–434–3575
Public university

Arizona

Northern Arizona University
Carl DeRosa, PT, Ph.D., Chairman
Dept. of PT
CU Box 15105
Northern Arizona University
Flagstaff, AZ   86011
520–523–4092
Public university

Arkansas

University of Central Arkansas
Venita Lovelace–Chandler, Ph.D., PT, PCS
Chairperson
Dept. of PT
University of Central Arkansas
201 Donaghey, HSC 200
Conway, AR   72035–0001
501–450–5548
Public university

California

California State University, Fresno
Darlene Stewart, PT, Chair
PT Program
CSU Fresno
2345 E. San Ramon
Fresno, CA   93740–0029
209–278–2022
Public university

California State University, Long Beach
Ray Morris, PT, Chairman
PT Dept.
College Of Health and Human Services
California State University, Long Beach
1250 Bellflower Blvd.
Long Beach, CA.   90840
310–985–4072
Public university

California State University, Northridge
Donna Redman–Bentley, Ph.D., PT Director
Dept. of Health Science, HLTH
Northridge, CA   91330
818–885–3101
Public university

Chapman University
Judith S. Canfield, Ed.D, PT, Director
School of Physical Therapy
Chapman University
333 North Glassell
Orange, CA   92666
714–997–6786
Private university

Loma Linda University
Larry Chinnock, MBA, PT, Director
Department of PT
School of Allied Health Professions
Loma Linda University
Loma Linda, CA   92350
909–824–4632
Private university

Mt. St. Marys College
Cynthia Moore Schwartz, MS, PT, Chair
Dept. of PT
Mount St. Marys College
12001 Chalon Rd.
Los Angeles, CA   90049
310–471–9519
Private college

Samuel Merritt College
Martha J. Jewell, Ph.D., PT, Chairperson
Dept. of PT
370 Hawthorne Ave.
Oakland, CA   94609
510–869–6241
Private college

College of Osteopathic Medicine of the Pacific
Elizabeth Rogers, Ed.D, PT
Chairperson
Dept. of PT
352 Pomona Mall East
Pomona, CA   91766–1889
909–469–5294
Private college

University of California/San Francisco State University
Nancy Byl, Ph.D., PT, Co–Director
Graduate Program in Physical Therapy
School of Medicine
Box 0736
University of California, San Francisco
San Francisco, CA   94143
415–476–3452
Public university

San Francisco State University
Ann Hallum, Ph.D., P.T., Co–Director
Graduate Program in Physical Therapy
San Francisco State University
1600 Holloway Avenue
San Francisco, CA   94132
415–338–2001
Public university

University of Southern California
Helen J. Hislop, Ph.D., PT, Professor and Chair
Dept. of Physical Therapy
University of Southern California
1540 East Alcazar Street CHP–155
Los Angeles, CA   90033
213–342–2900
Private university

University of the Pacific
J. Carolyn Hultgren, MPH, PT, Chairman
Dept. of PT
School of Pharmacy
University of the Pacific
Stockton, CA   95211
209–946–2886
Private university

Colorado

University of Colorado
Pauline Cerasoli, Ed.D, PT, Director
Physical Therapy Program
Health Science Center
4200 E. Ninth Ave. Box E244
Denver, Co.   80262
303–372–9144
Public university

Connecticut

Quinnipiac College
Edward Tantorski, MPH, PT, Program Director
Dept. of PT
School of Health Science
Quinnipiac College
Mt. Carmel Avenue
Hamden, CT.   06518
203–281–8681
Private college

The University of Connecticut
Pamela L. Roberts, MA, PT, Director
Program in Physical Therapy
School of Allied Health Professions
358 Mansfield Road
The University of Connecticut
Storrs, CT   06269–2101
203–486–0049
Public university

Delaware

University of Delaware
Paul Mettler, Ed.D, PT
Director
Physical Therapy Program
319 Mckinly Laboratory
University of Delaware
Newark, DE   19716
302–831–8910
Public university

District of Columbia

Howard University
Marilys Randolph, Ph.D., PT
Interim Chairperson
Dept. of PT
College of Allied Health Sciences
Howard University
6th and Bryant Street NW
Washington, DC   20059
202–806–7613/15
Private university

Florida

Barry University
Luis Vargas, Ph.D., PT
Director
11300 NE 2nd Ave.
Miami Shores, FL   33161–6695
305–899–3540
Private university

Florida A&M University
Keith R. Gaden, Ph.D., PT
Director
Division of Physical Therapy
Florida A&M University
School of Allied Health Sciences
Room 223 Ware–Rhancy Building
Tallahassee, FL   32307
904–599–3820
Public university

Florida International University
Awilda R. Haskins, PT, Ed.D
Chairperson
Dept. of PT
College of Health
Florida International University
Miami, FL   33199
305–348–2266
Public university

University of Central Florida
Gregory Frazer, Ph.D., Chair
Department of Physical Therapy
PO Box 160000 Trailer 544
University of Central Florida
Orlando, FL   32816–2200
407–823–3470
Public university

University of Florida
Denis Brunt, Ed.D, PT
Acting Chairman
Dept. of PT
College of Health Related Professions
University of Florida
Box 100154

Gainesville, FL   32610–0154
904–395–0085
Public university

University of Miami
Sherrill H Hays, Ph.D., PT
Director
Division of Physical Therapy
Dept. of Orthopedics and Rehabilitation
School of Medicine
University of Miami
5915 Ponce de Leon Blvd. 5th Fl
Coral Gables, FL   33146
305–284–4535
Private university

University of North Florida
Martha C. Rader, Ph.D., PT
Director, Physical Therapy Program
College of Health–Founders Hall
University of North Florida
4567 St. Johns Bluff Road S.
Jacksonville, FL   32224
904–646–2840
Public university

Georgia

Emory University
Pamela Catlin, Ed.D, PT, Director
Division of PT
Emory University
1441 Clifton Rd. NE
Atlanta, GA   30322
404–712–5657
Private university

Georgia State University
Barney LeVeau, PH.D., PT, Chairman
Dept. of PT
Georgia State University
University Plaza
Atlanta, GA   30303
404–651–3091
Public university

Medical College of Georgia
Jan F Perry, PH.D., PT, Chairman
Dept. of Physical Therapy
Medical College of Georgia
Augusta, GA   30912–0800
706–721–2141
Public university

North Georgia College
Lynda Woodruff, PH.D., PT, Director
Graduate Program in Physical Therapy
North Georgia College
Barnes Hall, Rm. A–6
Dahlonega, GA   30597
706–864–1422
Public College

Idaho

Idaho State University
Alexander G. Urfer, Ph.D., PT, Professor and Chair
Director
Department of Physical Therapy
Box 8002
Idaho State University

Pocatella, ID 83209
208–236–4095
Public university

Illinois

Bradley University
Mary Jo Mays, Ph.D., PT, Chairperson
Department of PT
Bradley University
1501 W Bradley Ave
Peoria, IL 61625
309–677–3489
Private university

Northern Illinois University
M.J. Blaschak, Ph.D., PT, Coordinator
Physical Therapy Program
School of Allied Health Professions
Northern Illinois University
Dekalb, IL   60115
815–753–1383 ext. 6243
Public university

Northwestern University
Sally C. Edelsberg, MS, PT, Director
Programs in PT
The Medical School
Northwestern University
645 North Michigan Avenue
Suite 1100
Chicago, IL   60611–2814
312–908–6786 ext. 8160
Private university

University of Health Sciences The Chicago Medical School
Elizabeth Coulson, MBA, PT, Chairman
Physical Therapy Program
School of Related Health Sciences
The Chicago Medical School /
Herman M. Finch University of Health Sciences
3333 Green Bay Road
North Chicago, IL   60064
708–578–3307
Private college

University of Illinois at Chicago
Jules Rothstein, Ph.D., PT, Head
Dept. of Physical Therapy
The University of Illinois at Chicago
1919 W Taylor St. M/C898
Chicago, IL   60612
312–996–7764/4350
Public university

Indiana

Indiana University
Constance McCloy, Ed.D, PT, Director
Physical Therapy Program
Indiana University
Ball Residence Hall, #112
1226 W. Michigan Street
Indianapolis, IN   46202–5180
317–278–1875
Public university

University of Evansville
Cheryl Giffith, MA, PT, Chairman
Dept. of PT

University of Evansville
1800 Lincoln Ave.
Evansville, IN   47722
812–479–2341
800–423–8633 ext. 2468 (admissions)
Private university

University of Indianapolis
Elizabeth Domholdt, Ed.D, PT, Dean
Krannert Graduate School of Physical Therapy
University of Indianapolis
1400 E. Hanna Ave.
Indianapolis, IN   46227–3697
317–788–3500
Private university

Iowa

The University of Iowa
David H. Nielson, Ph.D., PT
Director and Professor
Physical Therapy Graduate Program
College of Medicine
2600 Steindler Bldg.
The University of Iowa
Iowa City, IA   52242–1008
319–335–9791
Public university

University of Osteopathic Medicine and Health Sciences
M. Susan Cigelman, Ed.S., PT, Director
Physical Therapy Program
College of Health Sciences
University of Osteopathic Medicine and Health Sciences
3200 Grand Ave.
Des Moines, IA 50312
515–271–1634
Private Health Science University

Kansas

The University of Kansas Medical Center
Chukuka S Enwemeka, Ph.D., PT
Professor and Chairman
Dept. of Physical Therapy Education
3056 Robinson Hall
The University of Kansas Medical Center
3901 Rainbow Blvd.
Kansas City, KS   66160–7601
913–588–6799
Public university

Wichita State University
Linda Black, PT,
Interim Director
Dept. of PT
College of Health Professions
Wichita State University
Wichita, KS   67260–0043
316–689–3604
Public university

Kentucky

University of Kentucky Medical Center
Terry Malone, Ed.D, PT, Director
Physical Therapy Division
University of Kentucky Medical Center
Medical Center
Rm. 4, Annex I
Lexington, KY   40536–0079
606–323–5415
Public university

University of Louisville
Nancy Urbscheit, Ph.D., PT, Program Director
Physical Therapy Program
School of Allied Health Sciences
University of Louisville
Carmichael Building
525 E. Madison Street
Louisville, KY   40292
502–852–7815
Public university

Louisiana

Louisiana State University Medical Center
Joseph M. McCulloch, Jr., Ph.D., PT, Head
Department of Physical Therapy
School of Allied Health Professions
Louisiana State University Medical Center
PO Box 33932
Shreveport, LA   71130–3932
318–675–6820
504–568–4288 (New Orleans)
Public university

Maine

University of New England
Joyce MacKinnon, Ed.D, PT, Chair
Department of Physical Therapy
University of New England
11 Hills Beach Road
Biddeford, ME 04005
207–283–0171
Private university

Maryland

University of Maryland–Baltimore
Clarence W. Hardiman, Ph.D., PT, Chairman
Department of Physical Therapy
University of Maryland
School of Medicine
100 Penn Street, Room 115
Baltimore, MD   21201
410–706–7720
Public university

University of Maryland Eastern Shore
Raymond L. Blakely, Ph.D., PT, Director
Department of Physical Therapy
University of Maryland, Eastern Shore
Kiah Hall
Princess Anne, MD   21853
410–651–6301
Public university

Massachusetts

Boston University
Catherine Certo, Sc.D., PT, Program Director
Department of Physical Therapy
Sargent College of Allied Health Professions
Boston University
635 Commonwealth Avenue
Boston, MA   02215
617–353–2720
Private university

Northeastern University
Ann C. Noonan, Ed.D, PT, Acting Chair
Department of Physical Therapy
Rm. 6 Robinson Hall
Northeastern University
360 Huntington Avenue
Boston, MD   02115
617–373–3160
Private university

Simmons College
Diane Jette, MS, PT, Director
Graduate School for Health Studies
Graduate Program in Physical Therapy
Simmons College
300 The Fenway
Boston, MA   02115
617–521–2650
Private college

Springfield College
Linda J. Tsoumas, MS, PT, Chairman
Department of Physical Therapy
Springfield College
263 Alden Street
Springfield, MA   01109
413–748–3369
Private college

University of Massachusetts – Lowell
Joseph A. Dorsey, Ed.D, PT, Chairman
Program in Physical Therapy
University of Massachusetts – Lowell
Weed Hall
South Campus
Lowell, MA   01854
508–934–4517
Public university

Michigan

Andrews University
Wayne Perry, MBA, PT, Director
Department of Physical Therapy
Andrews University
Berrien Springs, MI   4910–0420
616–471–2878
800–827–AUPT
Private university

Grand Valley State University
Jane Toot, Ph.D., PT, Dept. Chair
Physical Therapy Department
Grand Valley State University

Allendale, MI   49401
616–895–3356
Public university

Oakland University
Beth Marcoux, Ph.D., PT, Director
Program in Physical Therapy
School of Health Sciences
Oakland University
Rochester, MI   48309–4401
810–370–4041
Public university

University of Michigan – Flint
Paulette Cebulski, Ph.D., PT, Director
Physical Therapy Department
School of Health Professions and Studies
University of Michigan – Flint
Flint, MI   48502–2186
810–762–3373
Public university

Wayne State University
Louise R. Amundsen, Ph.D., PT, Chair
Department of Physical Therapy
Wayne State University
Detroit, MI   48202
313–577–1432
Public university

Minnesota

The College of St. Catherine – Minneapolis
Debra Sellheim, MA, PT, Director
PT Program
The College of St. Catherine
601 25th Ave., South
Minneapolis, MN   55454
612–690–7828
Private college

Mayo School of Health Related Sciences
John P. Cummings, Ph.D., PT
Physical Therapy Program
Mayo School of Health Related Sciences
200 First Street, SW
Rochester, MN   55905
507–284–2054
Private college

The College of ST. Scholastica
Sandy Marden–Lokken, MA, PT, Chair
Department of Physical Therapy
The College of St. Scholastica
1200 Kenwood Avenue
Duluth, MN   55811
218–723–6786/6285
Private college

University of Minnesota
James R. Carey, Ph.D., PT, Director
Program in Physical Therapy
Box 388 UMHC
University of Minnesota
Minneapolis, MN   55455
612–626–5887
Public university

Mississippi

University of Mississippi Medical Center
Neva F. Greenwald, MSPH, PT
Chairman
Physical Therapy Department
School of Health Related Professions
University of Mississippi Medical Center
2500 N. State Street
Jackson, MS   39216
601–984–6330
Public university

Missouri

Maryville University
Joanna Schroer, Ph.D., PT, Program Director
Department of Physical Therapy
Maryville University
13550 Conway Road
St. Louis, MO   63141
314–576–9523
Private college

Rockhurst College
Ellen F. Spake, MS, PT, Chairman
Physical Therapy Education
Rockhurst College
1100 Rockhurst Road
Kansas City, MO   64110
816–926–4059
Private college

St. Louis University
Irma Ruebling, MA, PT, Chairman
Department of Physical Therapy
St. Louis University
1504 South Grand Blvd.
Room 306
St. Louis, MO   63104
314–577–8505
Private university

University of Missouri
Marilyn Sanford, Ph.D., PT, Director
Physical Therapy Program
School of Health Related Professions
University of Missouri – Columbia
106 Lewis Hall
Columbia, MO   65211
314–882–7103
Public university

Washington University
Susan S. Deusinger, Ph.D., PT, Director
Program in Physical Therapy
Washington University
School of Medicine
Campus Box 8502
4444 Forest Park Blvd., Suite 1101
St. Louis, MO   63108
314–286–1400
Private university

Montana

The University of Montana
Ann K. Williams, Ph.D., PT, Chair

Physical Therapy Program
The University of Montana
Missoula, MT   59812
406–243–4753
Public university

Nebraska

University of Nebraska Medical Center
Patricia Hageman Ph.D., PT, Director and Assistant Professor
Division of Physical Therapy Education
University of Nebraska College of Medicine
600 South 42nd
Box 984420
Omaha, NE   68198–4420
402–559–4259
Public university

New Jersey

Kean College of New Jersey
University of Medicine & Dentistry of New Jersey
Alma Merians, Ph.D., PT, Director
Physical Therapy Program
School of Health Related Professions
University of Medicine & Dentistry of New Jersey
65 Bergen Street
Newark, NJ   07107–3001
201–982–5272
Public university

Rutgers, The State University of New Jersey, Graduate School –
Camden/
University of Medicine & Dentistry of New Jersey
Marie R. Nardone, MS, PT, Program Director
Masters Physical Therapy Program
Rutgers, The State University of New Jersey Graduate Studies –
Camden/
University of Medicine & Dentistry of New Jersey
401 Haddon Avenue
Camden, NJ   08103–1506
609–964–2690
Public university

The Richard Stockton College of New Jersey
Bess Kathrins, MS, PT, Associate Professor and Director
Physical Therapy Program
The Richard Stockton State College of New Jersey
Jim Leeds Road
Pomona, NJ   08240
609–652–1776
Public university

New Mexico

University of New Mexico
Ronald Andrews, MS, PT, Director
Division of Physical Therapy
University of New Mexico
Room 204, Health Sciences & Services Building
Albuquerque, NM   87131
505–277–5755
Public university

New York

Columbia University
Joan Edelstein MA, PT, Director
Program in Physical Therapy
Columbia University
630 West 168th Street 3Ð458
New York, NY   10032
212–305–3781
Private university

D'Youville College
Susan Bennett, Ed.D, PT, Director
Physical Therapy Program
D'Youville College
One D'Youville Square
320 Porter Ave.
Buffalo, NY   14201–1084
716–881–7624
Private college

Daemen College
Richard Schweichler, PT, Program Director
Physical Therapy Department
Daemen College
4380 Main Street
Amherst, NY   14226
716–839–8345
Private college

Hunter College
Gary Krasilovsky, PH.D., PT, Assistant Professor and Director
Physical Therapy Program
School of Health Sciences
Hunter College
425 East 25th Street
New York, NY   10010
212–481–4469
Public College

Ithaca College
Winifred Mauser, ED.D, PT and Chair
Department of Physical Therapy
Ithaca College
Ithaca, NY   14850–7183
607–274–3124
Private college

Long Island University
William M. Susman, PH.D., PT, Associate Professor and Director
Division of Physical Therapy
Long Island University
University Plaza
Brooklyn, NY   11201
718–488–1063
Private university

New York University
Andrew L. McDonough, PT, Chairman
Physical Therapy Department
New York University
Weissman Building, 2nd Floor
345 E. 24th Street
New York, NY   10010Ð4086
212–998–9400
Private university

Russell Sage College
James Brennan, PT, Program Director
Department of Physical Therapy
Russell Sage College
Troy, NY   12180
518–270–2266
Private college

State University of New York at Buffalo
Susan Roehrig, PH.D., PT, Program Director
Physical Therapy Program
State University of New York at Buffalo
Department of Physical Therapy and Exercise Science
410 Kimball Tower – Main Street Campus
Buffalo, NY   14214
716–829–2941
Public university

State University of New York at Stony Brook
Richard Johnson, MD, PT
Department of Physical Therapy
School of Health Technology & Management
Health Science Center
State University of New York at Stony Brook
Stony Brook, NY   11794–8201
516–444–3250
Public university

State University of New York Health Science Center at Brooklyn
Joseph A. Balogun, PH.D., PT, Professor and Chairman
Physical Therapy Program
State University of New York Health Science Center at Brooklyn
450 Clarkson Avenue, Box 16
Brooklyn, NY   11203–2098
718–270–7720
Public Health Science College

State University of New York at Syracuse
Charles E. Meacci, ED.D, PT, Department Chairperson
Department of Physical Therapy
College of Health Related Professions
State University of New York Health Science Center at Syracuse
750 East Adams Street
Syracuse, NY   13210
315–464–5101
Public Health Science College

The College of Staten Island
Jeffrey Rotham, ED.D, PT
Program Director & Professor
Physical Therapy Program
The College of Staten Island
The City University of New York
2800 Victory Boulevard
Staten Island, NY   10314
718–982–3153

Touro College
Jill Auster–Liebhaber, MA, PT, Director
Physical Therapy Program
Barry Z. Levine School of Allied Health Sciences
Touro College
Building 10
135 Carman Road
Dix Hills, NY   11746
516–673–3200 ext. 220
Private college

North Carolina

Duke University
Robert C. Bartlett, MS, PT, Professor and Chairman

Graduate Program in Physical Therapy
Duke University
PO Box 3965
Durham, NC   27710
919–684–3135
Private university

East Carolina University
Bruce C. Albright, PH.D., PT, Chairperson
Department of Physical Therapy
East Carolina University
School of Allied Health Sciences
Greenville, NC   27858–4353
919–757–4450
Public university

University of North Carolina at Chapel Hill
Darlene K. Sekerak, PH.D., PT, Director
Division of Physical Therapy
University of North Carolina at Chapel Hill
Medical School Wing E 222H–CB #7135
Chapel Hill, NC   27599–7135
919–966–4709
Public university

Winston–Salem State University
Eddie L. Harden, MS, PT
Program Coordinator
Physical Therapy Program
Winston–Salem State University
601 Martin Luther King, Jr. Drive
Winston–Salem, NC   27110
910–750–2193–2190

North Dakota

University of North Dakota
Thomas M. Mohr, PT, PH.D., Professor and Chair
Department of Physical Therapy
School of Medicine
University of North Dakota
PO Box 9037
Grand Forks, ND   58202–9037
701–777–2831
Public university

Ohio

Cleveland State University
John J. Jeziorowski, PH.D., PT, ATC, Director
Physical Therapy Department
Department of Health Sciences
Cleveland State University
1983 East 24th Street, Fenn Tower 609
Cleveland, OH   44115
216–687–3567
Public university

Medical College of Ohio in Consortium with: 1) Bowling Green State
University and 2) The University of Toledo
Catherine Hornbeck, MS, PT, Director
Physical Therapy Program
Medical College of Ohio
2601 Ida Marie Dowling Hall
PO Box 10008
Toledo, OH   43699–0008
419–381–3518
Public university

Ohio State University
Stephen L. Wilson, PH.D., Acting Director
Division of Physical Therapy
Ohio State University
306 Allied Medical Professions
1583 Perry Street
Columbus, OH   43210
614–292–5921
Public university

Ohio University
Dennis C. Cade, PH.D., PT, Interim Director
School of Physical Therapy
Room 199 Convocation Center
Ohio University
Athens, OH   45701
614–593–1225
Public university

Oklahoma

Langston University
Denise Chapman, PH.D., PT, Program Director
Physical Therapy Program
School of Nursing & Health Professions
Langston University
Langston, OK   73050
405–466–3411
Public university

University of Oklahoma
Martha J. Ferretti, MPH, PT, Chairman
Department of Physical Therapy
College of Allied Health
Health Science Center
University of Oklahoma
PO Box 26901
Oklahoma City, OK   73190
405–271–2131
Public university

Oregon

Pacific University
Daiva Banaitis, PH.D., PT, Professor and Director
School of Physical Therapy
Pacific University
2043 College Way
Forest Grove, OR   97116
503–357–6151
Private university

Pennsylvania

Beaver College
Rebecca L. Craik, PH.D., PT, Chairman
Department of Physical Therapy
Beaver College
450 S. Easton Road
Glenside, Pa 19038Ð3295
215–572–2950
Private college

Duquesne University
Robert C. Morgan, PH.D., PT, Chairman

Department of Physical Therapy
School of Allied Health Sciences
Duquesne University
109 Health Sciences Building
Pittsburgh, PA   15282
412–396–5542
Private university

Gannon University
Kathleen A. Cegles, M.Ed., PT, Interim Program Director
Dept. of Physical Therapy
Gannon University
Villa Maria College of Health Sciences
University Square – AC 388
Erie, PA   16541–0001
814–871–5639
Private university

Medical College of Pennsylvania & Hahnemann University
Risa Granick, Ed.D, MPA   , PT, Interim Chair
Programs in Physical Therapy
Medical College of Pennsylvania & Hahnemann University
MS 502
201 North 15th Street
Philadelphia, PA   19102
215–762–1750/1758
Private university

Philadelphia College of Pharmacy and Science
Kevin A. Cody, Ph.D., PT, Chairman
Physical Therapy Program
Philadelphia College of Pharmacy and Science
600 South 43rd Street
Philadelphia, PA   19104
215–596–8810
Private university

Slippery Rock University
Jan K. Richardson, PT, Ph.D., OCS, Director
School of Physical Therapy
Slippery Rock University
Suite 100, North Rd.
Slippery Rock, PA   16057
412–738–2080
Public university

Temple University
Ann Van Sant, Ph.D., PT, Chairperson
Department of Physical Therapy
College of Allied Health Professions
Temple University
3307 North Broad Street
Philadelphia, PA   19140
215–707–4815/16
Public university

Thomas Jefferson University
Roger M. Nelson, Ph.D., PT, Professor and Chairman
Department of Physical Therapy
College of Allied Health Sciences
Thomas Jefferson University
EDISON 830
130 South 9th Street
Philadelphia, PA   19107
215–955–8025
Private university

University of Pittsburgh
Anthony Delitto, Ph.D., PT, Chairman
Department of Physical Therapy
101 Pennsylvania Hall
University of Pittsburgh
Pittsburgh, PA   15261

412–624–8990
Public university

University of Scranton
Carolyn E. Barnes, Ph.D., PT, Professor and Chairperson
Department of Physical Therapy
University of Scranton
800 Linden Street
Scranton, PA   18510–4586
717–941–7494
Private university

Puerto Rico

University of Puerto Rico
Carmen L. Colon, MA, PT, Acting Director
Physical Therapy Program
College of Health Related Professions
Medical Sciences Campus
University of Puerto Rico
GPO Box 365067
San Juan, PR   00936–5067
809–758–2525 EXT. 4200
Public university

Rhode Island

University of Rhode Island
Mark J. Rowinski, Ph.D., PT, Director
Physical Therapy Program
Independence Square II
The University of Rhode Island
Kingston, RI   02881–0180
401–792–5001
Public university

South Carolina

Medical University of South Carolina
Lisa K. Saladin, BMRPT, MSC   , Director
Physical Therapy Program
Medical University of South Carolina
171 Ashley Avenue
Charleston, SC   29425–2701
803–792–2961
Public university

South Dakota

University of South Dakota
Lana Svien, MA, PT, Acting Program Director
Department of Physical Therapy
University of South Dakota
414 E. Clark
Vermillion, SD   57069
605–677–5915
Public university

Tennessee

Tennessee State University
Dolly Swisher, MDiv, PT, CHT, Department Head
Physical Therapy Department
Tennessee State University
3500 John A. Merritt Boulevard
Nashville, TN   37209–1561
615–963–5881
Public university

The University of Tennessee at Chattanooga
Larry J. Tillman, Ph.D., Acting Department Head

Department of Physical Therapy
The University of Tennessee at Chattanooga
615 McCallie Avenue
Chattanooga, TN   37403–2598
615–755–4747
Public university

University of Tennessee
Barbara H. Connolly, Ed.D, PT, Associate Professor and Chairman
Department of Rehabilitation Sciences
University of Tennessee
822 Beale Street, 3rd Floor
Memphis, TN   38163
901–448–5888
Public university

Texas

Southwest Texas State University
Barbara Sanders, Ph.D., PT, Director
Physical Therapy Program
Southwest Texas State University
Health Science Center
601 University Drive
San Marcos, TX   78666
512–245–9351
Public university

Texas Tech University Health Science Center
H. H. Merrifield, Ph.D., PT, Chairman
Department of Physical Therapy
School of Allied Health
Texas Tech University Health Sciences Center
Lubbock, TX   79430
806–743–3226
Public university

Texas Woman's University
Carolyn Rozier, Ph.D., PT, Dean
School of Physical Therapy
Texas Woman's University
Box 22487, TWU Station
Denton, TX   76204–0487
817–898–2460
Dallas (214) 706–2300
Houston (713) 794–2070
Public university

US Army–Baylor University
Col Michael A. Smutok, Ph.D., PT, Director
Graduate Program in Physical Therapy
U.S. Army–Baylor University
Army Medical Specialist Corps Division
Academy of Health Sciences
U.S. Army
3151 Scott Road
Ft. Sam Houston, TX   78234–6138
502–626–0360
Public university

University of Texas Health Science Center at San Antonio
Ron Scott, JD, PT, Interim Chair
Department of Physical Therapy
University of Texas Health Science Center at San Antonio
7703 Floyd Curl Drive
San Antonio, TX   78284–7781
210–567–3151
Public university

University of Texas Medical Branch at Galveston
Kurt Mossberg, Ph.D., PT, Interim Chair
Department of Physical Therapy, J28
School of Allied Health Sciences

University of Texas Medical Branch at Galveston
301 University Boulevard
Galveston, TX   77555–1028
409–772–3068
Public Health Science University

University of Texas Southwestern Medical Center at Dallas
Patricia Winchester, Ph.D., PT, Chair
Department of Physical Therapy
School of Allied Health Sciences
University of Texas Southwestern Medical Center at Dallas
5323 Harry Hines Blvd.
Dallas, TX   75235
214–648–1550
Public Health Science College

Utah

University of Utah
R. Scott Ward, Ph.D., PT, Co–Director
Division of Physical Therapy
College of Health
1130 Annex, Wing B
University of Utah
Salt Lake City, UT   84112
801–581–8681
Public university

Vermont

University of Vermont
Samuel B. Feitelberg, PT, Chairperson
Department of Physical Therapy
School of Allied Health Sciences
University of Vermont
305 Rowell Bldg.
Burlington, VT   05405–0068
802–656–3252
Public university

Virginia

Old Dominion University
George Maihafer, Ph.D., PT, Associate Professor and Director
Program in Physical Therapy
School of Community Health Professions and Physical Therapy
Old Dominion University
Norfolk, VA   23529–0288
804–683–4409
Public university

Shenandoah University – Winchester Medical Center
Walter J. Personius, Ph.D., PT, Professor and Chairman
Program in Physical Therapy
Shenandoah University–Winchester Medical Center
333 West Cork Street
Winchester, VA   22601
800–432–2266
Private university

Virginia Commonwealth University
Robert L. Lamb, Ph.D., PT, Chairman
Department of Physical Therapy
Medical College of Virginia Campus

Virginia Commonwealth University
Box 980224
Richmond, VA   23298–0224
804–828–0234
Public university

Washington

Eastern Washington University
Walter H. Erikson, MS, PT, Chair
Department of Physical Therapy
526 Fifth Street, MS4
Eastern Washington University
Cheney, WA   99004–2431
509–458–6435
Public university

University of Puget Sound
Kathie Hummel–Berry, M.Ed., PT
Dept. Chair
School of Physical Therapy
University of Puget Sound
1500 North Warner
Tacoma, WA   98416
206–756–3281/3211
Private university

University of Washington
JoAnn McMillan, MS Ed., PT, Head
Division of Physical Therapy
Department of Rehabilitation Medicine RJ–30
University of Washington
Box 356490
Seattle, WA   98195–6490
206–685–7408
Public university

West Virginia

West Virginia University
Mary Beth Mandich, PH.D., PT, Interim Chairperson
Division of Physical Therapy
School of Medicine
West Virginia University
PO Box 9226
Morgantown, WV   26506–9226
304–293–3610
Public university

Wisconsin

Marquette University
Richard H. Jensen, PH.D., PT, Director
Program in Physical Therapy
Marquette University
PO Box 1881
Milwaukee, WI   53201–1881
414–288–7161
Private university

University of Wisconsin at La Crosse
Patricia A. Wilder, PH.D., PT, Associate Professor and Chair
Department of Physical Therapy
University of Wisconsin at LaCrosse
243 Cowley Hall
LaCrosse, WI   54601
608–785–8470
Public university

University of Wisconsin – Madison
Barbara J. Morgan, PH.D., PT, Coordinator

Physical Therapy Program
5175 Medical Sciences Center
University of Wisconsin – Madison
1300 University Avenue
Madison, WI   53706–1536
608–263–0013
Public university

Canada

McGill University
Edith Aston–McCrimmon, MScA, PT, Associate Director
Physical Therapy Program
McGill University
3654 Drummond Street
Montreal, Quebec
Canada H3G1Y5
514–398–4500
Public university

Developing Programs

Master's Degree

Institute of Physical Therapy	St. Augustine, FL
Nova Southeastern University	North Miami Beach, FL
St. Ambrose University	Davenport, IA
Central Michigan University	Mt. Pleasant, MI
Andrews University/Dayton	Dayton, OH
Chatham College	Pittsburgh, PA
College Misericordia	Dallas, PA
Widener University	Chester, PA
Wheeling Jesuit College	Wheeling, WV
Concordia University Wisconsin	Mequon, WI

Doctoral Degree

Creighton University   Omaha, NE

**** For an updated list of developing programs or newly developing programs call 1–800–999–APTA.

Master's Programs

The University of Alabama Birmingham	GRE
Northern Arizona University	
University of Central Arkansas	
California State University, Fresno	
Chapman University	
Loma Linda University	GRE/AHPAT
Mount St. Mary's College	GRE
Samuel Merritt College	GRE
College of Osteopathic Medicine of the Pacific	
University of California, San Francisco/	
San Francisco State University	GRE
University of Southern California	GRE
University of the Pacific	GRE
University of Colorado	GRE
University of Delaware	
Barry University	
University of Miami	GRE
Emory University	GRE

North Georgia College	GRE
Idaho State University	GRE
Northwestern University	GRE
University of Evansville	
University of Indianapolis	GRE
The University of Iowa	GRE
University of Osteopathic Medicine & Health Sciences	
The University of Kansas Medical Center	GRE
Wichita State University	
University of Maryland Eastern Shore	
University of Maryland, Baltimore	
Boston University	GRE
Simmons University	
Springfield College	
University of Massachusetts–Lowell	GRE
Andrews University	
Grand Valley State University	
Oakland University	AHPAT
University of Michigan–Flint	
Mayo School of Health Related Sciences	GRE
The College of St. Scholastica	
College of St. Catherine–Minneapolis	
Rockhurst College	
St. Louis University	
Washington University	GRE
University of Nebraska Medical Center	
Rutgers, The State University of New Jersey	GRE

Columbia University	
D'Youville College	SAT
Ithaca College	SAT/ACT
Long Island University	
State University of New York at Syracuse	
The College of Staten Island	
Touro College	
Duke University	GRE
University of North Carolina–Chapel Hill	
University of North Dakota	
Ohio University	
Pacific University	
Beaver College	GRE
Duquesne University	
Gannon University	
Medical College of Pennsylvania &	GRE
Hahnemann University	
Philadelphia College of Pharmacy and Science	
Slippery Rock University	GRE
Temple University	GRE
Thomas Jefferson University	
University of Pittsburgh	GRE
University of Scranton	SAT
The University of Rhode Island	GRE
The University of South Dakota	GRE
Texas Woman's University	GRE
Texas Tech University Health Science Center	

University of Texas Galveston	AHPAT
US Army–Baylor University	GRE
Old Dominion University	GRE
Shenandoah University	GRE/SAT
Virginia Commonwealth University	
University of Puget Sound	
Marquette University	AHPAT

Bachelor's Programs

University of South Alabama	
University of Central Arkansas	
California State University, Fresno	
California State University, Northridge	
California State University at Long Beach	
Quinnipiac College	
The University of Connecticut	
Howard University	
Florida Agricultural And Mechanical University	
Florida International University	
University of Central Florida	
University of Florida	AHPAT
University of North Florida	
Georgia State University	
Medical College of Georgia	SAT
Bradley University	
Northern Illinois University	

University of Health Sciences The Chicago Medical School
University of Illinois at Chicago
Indiana University
University of Kentucky
University of Louisville
Louisiana State University
University of New England   SAT
Northeastern University   SAT
Wayne State University
University of Minnesota
University of Mississippi Medical Center
Maryville University   ACT
University of Missouri Ð Columbia
The University of Montana
Kean College of New Jersey
The Richard Stockton College of New Jersey
University of New Mexico
Daemen College
Hunter College
New York University
Russell Sage College
State University of New York at Buffalo
State University NY Stony Brook   AHPAT
State University of New York Brooklyn   GRE/AHPAT
State University of New York Health Science Center at Syracuse
East Carolina University
Winston–Salem State University

Cleveland State University

Medical College of Ohio

Ohio State University

Ohio University

Langston University

University of Oklahoma

University of Puerto Rico

Medical University of South Carolina   SAT

Tennessee State University

University of Tennessee

University of Tennessee/Chattanooga

Southwest Texas State University

University of Texas Southwestern Medical Center at Dallas

University of Texas Health Science Center San Antonio
APHAT

University of Utah

University of Vermont   SAT

Eastern Washington University

University of Washington   AHPAT

West Virginia University   AHPAT

University of Wisconsin - Madison

University of Wisconsin at LaCrosse

McGill University

Epilogue

Becoming a Physical Therapist is not an easy task. The road to success is a long and arduous one. Beginning in high school with a sound foundation of courses and study habits will make this a much easier and pleasant journey.

To fully appreciate the dilemma of a Physical Therapy school, put yourself, for a moment, in the shoes of the admissions officer at one of these schools. How do you determine which of those 500 applications for your program will provide you with the student who will make the best Physical Therapist? Do you go strictly by grades? Do you eliminate the student who has a wealth of experience already in the field, is empathetic, has life experiences which span cultures, but does not have the GPA of another student who is also applying? Do you eliminate the student with a 3.8 GPA in favor of the student with a 3.4 GPA because this student speaks better in a twenty-minute interview? Is there a way to determine in an individual has that rare combination of intelligence and empathy? Until these issues are settled within the profession of teaching Physical Therapy, books such as this one will be in great demand.

Both of the authors applied several different times to Physical Therapy Programs. We checked our mailboxes two to three times daily just as you will. The secret to our success in attaining our goal of attending Physical Therapy School was not in any secret formula. Hard work and sacrifice, renewed following rejection, was the key.

If you are reading this book you have already begun the journey. Good luck. In spite of the hardship and long hours of study in undergraduate school, the process of selling yourself to a school, followed by more long hours of study if accepted, the trip is worth it. Physical Therapy is a great profession that will provide you with a great sense of satisfaction and accomplishment. Stay the course, you will be glad you did.

ABOUT THE AUTHORS

SKIP HUNTER, P.T., A.T.,C.
Skip Hunter received a B.S. degree in Physical Therapy from the Medical University of South Carolina in 1978. In addition, he received certification as an athletic trainer by the National Athletic Trainers Association in 1978. He currently is Director of Sports Medicine for the Clemson Sports Medicine and Rehabilitation Center at 1007 Tiger Blvd., Clemson, SC. Before joining the Clemson Sports Medicine and Rehabilitation Center, he was Director of Sports Medicine at The Charlotte Sports Medicine Center for three years. Prior to this, he was trainer for the University of North Carolina at Chapel Hill football program for 8 years, 3 years as assistant and 5 years as head trainer. In addition, he served as trainer for field hockey, wrestling, tennis, track, and gymnastics. In 1989 and 1991 Hunter served as trainer for the US Soccer program with their under-twenty-one team in France and the World Cup team versus Trinidad in the U.S. He also served as the head trainer for the Charlotte Rage Arena football team in 1991.

Mr. Hunter teaches continuing education courses throughout the country, and has had numerous articles published in a variety of publications including The National Athletic Trainers Journal, The Physician and Sportsmedicine, The Journal of Orthopedics and Sports Physical Therapy, and The Journal of the American Physical Therapy Association. He is the co-author of *Orthotics for Sport and Therapy*. He is a member of the Sports Medicine Section of the American Physical Therapy Association and the National Athletic Trainers Association.

LORI WHITLOW
Lori Whitlow is a Certified Recreational Therapist. She received her B.S. degree from Clemson University in 1991. Ms. Whitlow has worked in Physical and Recreational Therapy since 1990. She has experience in many of the specialties of Physical Therapy such as Orthopedics, Geriatrics, and Rehabilitation. She has applied to Physical Therapy school over the past several years. Her experience in Physical Therapy as well as her applications to Physical Therapy school give her insight into the process of becoming a Physical Therapist.

Currently Ms. Whitlow is a Physical Therapy student at Wheeling Jesuit College in Wheeling, West Virginia.

Order Form

Please send _____ copies of *How To Become A Physical Therapist*.
ISBN 0-9649873-0-9.

(Quantity)   @ $19.95 = _____ _____

Total   _____

Make checks payable to SHE (Skip Hunter Enterprises, Inc.)

Signature:_____

Name:_____

Address:_____

City:_____ State:_____ Zip:_____

Send payment with order form to:

SHE   (Skip Hunter Enterprises, Inc.)
PO Box 61
Clemson, SC   29633

Please allow 4–6 weeks for delivery.